Contents

Introduction

Want a simple and sustainable way to shred fat, build muscle, increase your energy and feel like a new man? And do you want an approach that delivers the results at a massively accelerated rate and doesn't involve dieting?

Well, let me introduce Intermittent Fasting - the most sustainable and easy to adopt fitness hack that will get you in the best shape of your life.

Intermittent Fasting has exploded in popularity over the past year as the benefits and results it delivers become clear. It is used and loved by celebrities such as Hugh Jackman, Beyoncé, Benedict Cumerbatch and Ben Affleck.

But what is Intermittent Fasting?

Well, it is not a diet - it is a new approach to eating.

Intermittent Fasting is the process of cycling periods in which you eat with periods that you don't eat. These short fasting windows cause your body to produce a multitude of hormonal responses. These responses produce incredible benefits and results.

But what are the benefits? Well, here's a few examples...

- Shred fat (without dieting or limiting the foods you can eat)

- Build lean muscle rapidly

- Increased energy levels

- Heightened testosterone and growth hormone production

- Improvement to cognitive functioning

Fasting is the most powerful way to get in shape and become healthy because it is based on scientific evidence not "bro-science."

If you've ever tried to get in shape before and failed don't despair. The problem with most diets is that they put too many limitations on what you can eat. Intermittent fasting is the opposite of this – you don't need to make any changes to your diet to reap the rewards.

So what are you waiting for? Dive into the book now and learn everything you need to know about Intermittent Fasting – I take you through every single step and give you a simple, easy to follow guide.

What is Intermittent Fasting

Intermittent Fasting is a style of eating and an incredibly effective way to achieve a huge variety of fitness and health goals. It doesn't matter if you want to lose fat, build muscle, increase intelligence, increase testosterone, live longer or just save time and money- Intermittent Fasting will ensure you achieve it.

I prefer to not classify intermittent fasting as a diet, but rather a lifestyle. You will understand why as you read through this book.

Intermittent fasting (IF) is the practice of switching back and forth between predetermined periods in which you eat and periods in which you don't eat.

When most people hear this concept they disregard it and assume it sounds to complex or that they wouldn't be able to manage it. Some of the common things I often hear are:

"What the hell… not eating? I will go into starvation mode!"

"But I have to keep my metabolic fire stoked and burning to lose fat!"

"You're stupid Peter… there is no way that's healthy."

However these people forget that every single day of their lives they have been practicing intermittent fasting on some level. What do I mean by this? Well, when you sleep you fast and when you're awake you eat – this is intermittent fasting. These people are often usually undereducated on the topic and haven't studied just how beneficial it is.

The fitness industries approach to IF just takes this further by increasing the window of fasting and decreasing the window of eating.

At its core level the practice of intermittent fasting is very simple - do not let this fool you though as once you explore the area deeper it becomes highly complex. In this book I will take the complex data, scientific results and theories and break it all down into a simple, easy to understand format.

In the past years IF has become increasing popular gaining raving endorsements from bodybuilders, models, athletes and celebrities such as Hugh Jackman and Beyoncé. This explosion in popularity of IF is in no way surprising as once you start your IF journey you will see an incredible array of results.

The increasing popularity of IF is, in my mind, due to two main factors:

- The extensive list of powerful benefits it delivers (discussed in an upcoming chapter)

And;

- The ease of which it can be adopted and maintained.

It has been shown that most diets and dieters fail because of two main barriers.

These barriers are the complexity of managing a diet and the time they take to show results. How often have you heard someone wondering if "eating this food will negatively affect my diet" or "I've been on diet XYZ for 2 weeks now and I'm not seeing the results I want!"

Intermittent fasting knocks clean through these barriers with its simple, easy to follow procedures and its speed of results.

The concept of IF goes against much of what the fitness and health industry has long believed but as this book will detail – just because something is popular and repeated by everyone and their grandma's it doesn't mean it's true.

Common Fitness and Nutrition Myths

In the early days of its arising intermittent fasting came under a huge amount of scrutiny as it goes against everything that has been taught in the fitness industry for the past 50 years.

The concept of purposefully not eating is, at first appearances, a fitness fallacy. However once you explore the idea and challenge the past assumptions with scientific data you begin to see some shocking things.

I first off want to explore and debunk possibly the most well-known and quoted dietary "fact". This "fact" stands in the way of many people accepting the benefits of IF and is often quoted when criticising IF.

1. *"You have to eat 5-6 small meals a day to keep your metabolism burning."*

Unless you have lived under a rock for the past two decades I'm sure you've heard this from absolutely everyone. It is one of those rare pieces of advice that spreads like wildfire and is adopted by every-single-person. This advice has become so popular it has basically been adopted as a rock-solid fact.

However it is a lie, with zero scientific evidence to support it. That's right, one of the most well-known pieces of fitness and health advice is false.

The logic behind this theory is that eating small meals continually throughout the day will cause you to burn more fat. This comes from the idea that as eating increases your metabolic rate, eating frequently will keep your metabolic rate increased. Unfortunately this has never been proven, despite the fact that many studies have tried – and failed.

As is always the case with scientific research whilst some groups are trying to prove a theory, others are trying to disprove it. For this theory of frequent feeding, the teams disproving it won and multiple papers have been published on the topic. The most famous of which is a paper entitled:

"Increased Meal Frequency Does Not Promote Greater Weight Loss."

A team of Canadian researchers disproved the model of frequent feeding and detailed that it doesn't actually matter when or how often you eat, rather it is the amount you eat.

I want to note here that you can lose weight eating 6 small meals but it is not the frequency of eating or the meal timing that is the weight loss driver. Instead it is the amount you eat – small meals usually result in lower caloric intake.

Now for another piece of nutritional and fitness advice that has been touted by everyone for many years…

2. *"Breakfast is the Most Important Meal of the Day"*

This seemingly makes perfect sense and does have some inherent benefits to it, however it is not necessarily true and there is scores of evidence to disprove it. I am not saying breakfast is bad, wrong or that you should avoid it… I am simply noting that just because it is popular doesn't make it right and that there are more effective strategies.

The concept of breakfast being the most important meal of the day is that it helps you start the day, gives you energy and fuels your day. Now while these points have value to them, you have to remember most people make poor dietary choices at breakfast. These choices actually result in the opposite of the touted benefits occurring.

Combined with this is the idea that eating food (particularly carbohydrates) later in the evening will cause you to gain fat - this is another common myth that science has disproven. In actuality later feeding can result in some of the following benefits: increase in fat loss, increase in testosterone, better sleep and an increase in muscle gain.

There are benefits to not eating later in the evening but the evidence points to the benefits of eating later as outweighing the benefits of eating earlier.

Practisers of IF usually suggest skipping breakfast, I will explore this in more detail later.

3. *"Eat THIS, not that!"*

Another fitness and nutritional staple is that you must eat certain foods and follow a specific diet in order to achieve your goals.

Whether your goals are weight loss, gaining muscle or living a longer and healthier life every guru, nutritionist and personal trainer will espouse his or her preferred diet as the ONLY way to achieve your goals.

Some of the common diets you may have been told to follow are:

- Low carb, high protein, zero fat
- High Fat, high protein zero carb
- Slow-carb diet
- DASH diet
- Palaeolithic
- Carb cycling
- Atkins

There are literally hundreds of different diets you could follow, each of them have pros and cons but what I often find is that they all fall short in one area – how easy it is to stick to them.

Sure each of these diets will help you achieve your goals but no matter how effective a diet is, if you don't stick to it religiously you will negatively impact your progress. When you lock yourself into a specific diet you limit your choices and make it very hard to follow it – this results in failed dieting.

Intermittent fasting will circumvent this as it doesn't promote any particular diet style, instead it suggests a change in your eating frequency and window. Yes, there are some guidelines to follow but these are very loose and for the most part you can eat whatever type of foods you like.

The Benefits of Intermittent Fasting

So far I have alluded to some of the benefits intermittent fasting deliver but I haven't went into more detail. In this section I want to explore the range of awesome benefits that intermittent fasting will deliver to you. Firstly I will list off all the benefits in a bullet point fashion before going on to explain them in more detail.

IF has a huge number of benefits not only for your body composition but also for your mind and social life. So, what are the benefits?

Physiological Benefits

- Rapid Fat Loss

- Increase in Testosterone and HGH Production

- Lean Muscle Gain

- Increased Energy Levels

- Ability to Easily Control Hunger

- Higher Sex Drive

- Improvement to Hair and Skin

- Longevity of Life

Psychological and Lifestyle Benefits

- Improvement to Cognitive Abilities

- Better Sleep

- Save Time and Money

- Easy to Follow

- Reduction in Stress

So as you can see intermittent fasting has a whole host of awesome benefits which make it the perfect way to lose fat, build muscle and feel awesome. Now I want to dig a little deeper into some of the key benefits and explain the research and science behind them.

One of the main drivers behind IF's ability to rapidly burn fat is that when there is no food in the body (fasted state) your body will starting attacking its fat reserves to provide energy.

Placing your body in a fasted state will also cause a number of hormonal reactions to take place. One of the main reactions is that your body will begin to secrete a hugely increased amount of both growth hormone and testosterone. How much is a huge increase? Well one study found that a fast increased growth hormone production by 2000% in men.

These hormones are hugely important in the body and an increased production of them massively aids fat burning and muscle gain. Growth hormone is often referred to as "the fat burning hormone" and increased levels of testosterone have time and time again been linked with an accelerated amount of fat loss.

Additionally when you combine an increase in GH and testosterone production with a weight lifting routine you will add lean muscle at an accelerated rate. This is awesome for two main reasons: you build muscle rapidly and muscle raises your metabolic rate, meaning you burn additional fat.

Increased testosterone is also strongly linked to a reduction in stress, an increase in cognitive functioning, improvements to sleep and hugely spiked energy levels.

Looking at the other reactions that take place when your body is fasted it has been shown that intermittent fasting will decrease your insulin levels. This is important as insulin prevents lipolysis (the release of body fat stores). Without lipolysis occurring the body can't target its fat stores for energy. As a fast will blunt and lower insulin production it means your body can attack the fat stores – this both provides you with energy and helps you lose weight.

People are often worried that fasting will result in muscle loss as they think their body will attack muscle for energy - don't worry about this happening, it is a misconception about how the body works. The blunting of insulin production combined with the increase in hormones means that you are able to increase muscle whilst burning fat.

Another couple of points I want to elaborate on is that fasting also decreases the production of the hormone ghrelin. This is the hormone that influences your feelings of hunger and satiety. If you've ever had a hunger pang then ghrelin was being produced in higher amounts. Being in a fasted state blunts this, effectively preventing you from feeling as hungry as you might expect when fasting.

As I mentioned earlier in the book fasting is not a diet, rather it is a style of eating. For me this is one of the most crucial benefits as it makes it easy to adhere to, suitable for any lifestyle and gives you the ability to reap all its powerful benefits without interfering with your social life.

Diets can be very effective, when followed religiously, this however if often difficult as so many foods are off limits. Ever been out with friends for dinner when on a diet? Choosing something on the menu is stupidly difficult.

Intermittent fasting removes this as the benefits do not come from the foods you eat, instead they come from the physiological reactions that occur. Of course if you follow certain eating guidelines (discussed later) you will see accelerated results, but the key point is you do not have to eat the same meals over and over again.

Within the world of IF there exists various practices you can adopt. Each style has its pros and cons but they all deliver the benefits that were mentioned in the previous chapter. The effectiveness of the benefits will only vary slightly between each option so the most important thing is to pick a style that best suits your lifestyle.

All of the styles of IF revolve around the same basic concept: a large fasting window with a small eating window. The most common eating/fasting windows are listed below.

16/8 Split. Each day consists of a 16 hour fast followed by an 8 hour eating window.

This is the easiest to adopt and what I suggest for beginners. Considering that you will be sleeping for close to half of this fast makes it very easy to adopt.

18/6 Split. Each day consists of an 18 hour fast followed by a 6 hour eating window.

At 18 hours the effectiveness of fasting jumps massively and you will see accelerated results from the 16 hour window. I suggest adopting this after you have experimented with the 16/8 split.

20/4 Split. Each day consists of a 20 hour fast followed by a 4 hour eating window.

I find that this is a very, very effective window but due to the fact it is a daily 20 hour fast the impact it can be quite difficult to work around.

24 Hour Fast. Carried out twice per week.

This is not for beginners, once you have experimented with different fasting windows feel free to switch to this but do not attempt it as a beginner. Beginners attempting 24 hour fasts have not yet acclimatized their bodies to fasting and as a result will often fail.

36 Hour Fast. Once every 8-10 days.

For well-practiced intermittent fasters only. A 36 hour fast will be a mental struggle to get through, the benefits of it are huge but it is difficult to complete and difficult to work into a lifestyle. Do not ever go over 36 hours as your body will have burnt through all its fat stores and begin attacking muscle for energy.

The eating/fasting window that you eventually choose will not hugely impact your goals as each option will deliver the desired benefits. That said, what is important is the consistency in which you stick to your chosen option.

Don't treat it as something you can just randomly do when you feel like it, in order to get the results and benefits you must consistently follow your eating fasting window.

I want to mention that you do not need to stick to the exact same eating and fasting window every day of the week - but it does make it much easier to adhere to.

Intermittent Fasting and Food

I mentioned at the beginning of this book that IF is not a diet but a lifestyle choice. In this chapter I want to explore that concept further.

Firstly let's look at what a diet is as defined by the dictionary.

"A particular selection of food, as designed or prescribed to improve a person's physical condition… Such a selection or a limitation on the amount a person eats for reducing weight…The foods eaten, by a particular person or group."

Reading through those sentences all I can see is limitations – this is the problem with diets in my mind. They place too many limitations on the foods you can eat, the amount you can and make everything more confusing than it has to be.

Now I want to emphasise that diets can be very effective, however I tend to see them as useful for only very specific goals (such as getting to single digit body fat %) or for medical reasons.

For the majority of people though diets are not effective, they do not deliver the required results and they have a massive fall-out/failure rate.

This is because diets are limiting.

Intermittent fasting is not limiting. It is freeing.

IF frees you from all the technical details that diets have. If you begin to practice IF you will not have to adhere to the incredibly strict rules of diets. Instead you can eat whatever you want (within reason) and you can eat much more (again within reason).

I say within reason as if you eat fast food every single day and eat stupidly large portions then no drug, fitness routine or supplement is going to allow you to lose fat and be lean. Not to mention that fast foods are detrimental to your health, hormones, brain and internal organs. But back to what I was saying....

Intermittent fasting differs from dieting as you are not held in shackles by the rules of the diet. Want to eat white carbs? Go ahead! Want to have a pizza for a treat tonight? Go ahead! Don't want to change your current eating style? Well IF is the answer.

Due to the fact that the body reaps the majority of IF's benefits from the hormonal reactions that occur when you are in a fasted state it smashes the shackles that most diets place on you. As long as you place your body into a fasted state for at least 16 hours per day you will reap the rewards of IF.

If you are interested in stepping it up a notch and seeing highly accelerated results and more powerful benefits then there are certain eating choices you can make.

Accelerate Your Results Through Food

As I mentioned the main benefits of IF come from the hormonal reactions that occur when your body is in a fasted state. However you can achieve accelerated results by switching out your current eating style and following a few principles. Following these guidelines and principles will accelerate your results as you will eat foods that:

- Boost testosterone and growth hormone production

- Help burn fat

- Reduce insulin spikes

- Aid muscle growth

- Improve cognitive functioning

So if you are looking for accelerated results here are the guidelines that I would follow.

- Avoid processed and manufactured foods

- Avoid white carbohydrates

- Increase amount of protein in diet

- Increase amount of healthy fat in diet (olive oil, avocado etc.)

- Ensure 80% of your carbs come from legumes and beans

- Ensure the other 20% of your carbs come from whole-grains and whole-wheat's

- Eat green vegetables with every meal

- Use the following for seasoning: Garlic, paprika, cayenne, chilli flakes, black pepper and sea salt

- Reduce fruit intake, limit to one piece per day

- Drink only black coffee, herbal teas and water

Again, you don't have to stick to these guidelines but if you do you will see results and benefits at an accelerated rate.

If you want more details, a shopping list and recipe ideas I have put together 2 Free Gifts for you. Go check the gifts out by visiting www.goodlivingpublishing.com/fasting

Now you've read everything about IF and you understand how powerful it can be - it is time to get started.

Instead of just diving into fasting though I suggest you read this chapter. I'm going to suggest a few steps you take before you start practicing IF. Following the information here will help you in developing a plan, sticking to the plan and ultimately getting the awesome results you want.

So, what are the steps?

1. Decide a Starting Date.

I would highly recommend starting on a Monday, it just makes more sense. Pick a day and then follow the next few steps to be fully prepared for the starting time.

2. Choose a Fasting/Eating Split

Decide which eating and fasting window you want to adopt, again for beginners I always suggest the 16/8 as it is very easy to get used to and won't prove too difficult on your first attempt. Pick your window and then decide when you are going to stop eating the night before the fast – this will serve as your split and for the first week I suggest following it religiously. Once you've been practicing IF for a few weeks switching windows and times will become second nature to you, but for week 1 it's best to stick to the same times. So if you decide to stop eating at 9pm on the Sunday then you won't eat until 1pm on the Monday. After that 1-9pm will be your eating window.

3. Have a Cheat Day

The day before your first fast have a cheat day - eat a lot and eat whatever you want. This will serve two purposes for you. Firstly the more food you have in your system the easier the first fast will be. Secondly if you eat whatever you want the day before it means you won't crave these foods during the week.

4. Tell People

I highly suggest telling those who are closest to you about the new practice you are adopting. Explain why you are doing it and that you are committed – politely let them know you won't be eating at certain times and that you would love their support. By telling people in advance you will offset the chances of them offering you foods when you are fasted. One of the hardest challenges you will face is friends, family and colleagues offering you food – circumvent this by letting them know about your IF.

5. Buy Branch Chain Amino Acids (optional)

Branch Chain Amino Acids (BCAAs) can be very useful when fasting – they are a pure form of protein and are unbelievably powerful if you are doing longer fasts. Consuming 10g of BCAAs will help curb hunger without breaking your fast. Do not take more than 10g at a time but feel free to have two servings during your fast. If you are going to be exercising then I would highly suggest BCAAs.

6. Decide if You Are Going to Train

I will discuss fitness training and IF in the next chapter but decide if you are going to adopt or continue with a fitness routine whilst practicing IF. I do highly suggest it (explained in next chapter) but would say buy BCAAs if you are going to be training.

7. Start

Hell yeah!

Training and Intermittent Fasting

In order to reap the benefits of intermittent fasting you do not need to exercise. However if you choose to exercise you will see results on an unprecedented level.

As discussed earlier in the book IF will boost growth hormone and testosterone production as well as attacking fat cells and stores. Now if you add in an exercise routine (I suggest weight training) to this then the results you will see are incredible.

By adopting a weight training routine combined with your elevated hormones you will be able to add lean muscle faster than you thought was possible. Not to mention that the act of lifting weights also increases testosterone and growth hormone production, so your body will be getting a double dose of hormone production.

Weight training is also highly metabolic so you will shred the fat from your body and remember as I said earlier more muscle = less fat.

I also want to quickly mention that weight training and exercise is arguably the most effective way to protect your body from everything the world throws at you. It has been proven to reduce stress, help with depression, increase energy level, improve mental functioning, increase your happiness, better your life and help you live longer.

So, I do highly suggest you start to exercise and if you don't have a gym that's fine – bodyweight exercises such as push ups, air squats, lunges etc. will all aid you in your journey.

One final point I would like to add is that if you can train fasted – then do that. I understand it might not be possible for everyone due to scheduling but a way to upgrade your IF is to train fasted and then break your fast with a post workout meal.

Never go more than 2 hours after weight training without eating as your muscles will begin to breakdown and this will negatively impact your goals.

And on the topic of eating…

A Taster of the Recipes in Your Free Gift

As my way of saying "thank you" to you for buying my book I put together two free gifts for you:

"The Intermittent Fasting Recipe Book"

And

"The Intermittent Fasting Shopping List"

If you want to download your free gifts just head over to the following website:

www.GoodLivingPublishing.com/fasting

In this chapter of the book I'm going to give you a few sample recipes - it lets you get a taster of how awesome your free gift is. I've given you a sample of a breakfast, lunch and dinner recipe.

Ingredients

2 Large tomatoes, tops cut off and inside scooped out.

2 Rashers of bacon

Ground paprika, to taste

Sea salt, to taste

Directions

Preheat oven to 350F

Cook the bacon under a grill/broiler and once cooked remove and tear into small pieces.

Add the scooped tomato and bacon to a bowl along with paprika and mix well.

Spoon the mixture into the tomatoes and set on a baking tray.

Bake for 10-15 minutes.

Sprinkle salt to taste.

Ingredients

1 can of black beans, drained

3 tablespoons tomato paste

Ground paprika, to taste

Ground cayenne, to taste

1 whole-wheat tortilla

1 cup of shredded lettuce

¼ cup hot salsa

Directions

Add the shredded lettuce to a pot of water and bring to the boil.

Cover and let simmer until cooked, 5 minutes or so. Drain once cooked.

Place a pan over a medium heat and add the black beans, tomato paste, paprika, cayenne and salsa. Mix well and stir frequently.

Cook for 5 minutes.

Warm the tortilla in the microwave for 10 seconds.

Add the lettuce and black bean mix to the tortilla and wrap up.

Ingredients

1 salmon fillet

3 tablespoons sweet chilli sauce

1 red onion, chopped

1 garlic clove, finely chopped

1 courgette, sliced lengthwise

Directions

Preheat oven to 350F

Layer the bottom of an oven proof dish with chopped onion, garlic and courgette.

Place the salmon fillet on top and drizzle sweet chilli sauce over everything.

Cover and bake for 15-20 minutes.

Serve with green vegetables.

Conclusion

I hope you've enjoyed this book and are ready to get started with your intermittent fasting lifestyle. Just remember, I'm here with you on your journey so if you ever want to shoot me a question then don't hesitate to ask – I'm happy to help.

I'm going to close the book with a "quick guide to IF" so that you can check the bullet points if you ever need to jog your memory.

Thanks for reading.

Quick Guide to IF

- Choose a fasting/eating window and stick to it. 16/8 is easiest but I suggest 18/6

- Make sure your window suits your schedule

- For accelerated results follow the dietary suggestions of eating whole and natural foods with a high level of protein

- Train with heavy weights 3-4x per week and train fasted if possible

- Remember it is not a diet but a lifestyle

- Become awesome

Enjoy this book?

Please leave a review and let others know what you liked about this book?

Reviews are so crucial to self-published authors like myself and it would mean the world to me if you could leave me a quick review. Even one sentence would make a huge difference to me!

Thanks,

Peter

Other Books by Peter

<u>Naturally Triple Your Testosterone: A Guide to Hacking Your Hormones and Becoming Superhuman</u>

<u>The 6 Pack Chef: Easy to Cook, Delicious Recipes to Get Shredded and Reveal Your Abs</u>